CANDIDA DIET COOKBOOK FOR VEGANS

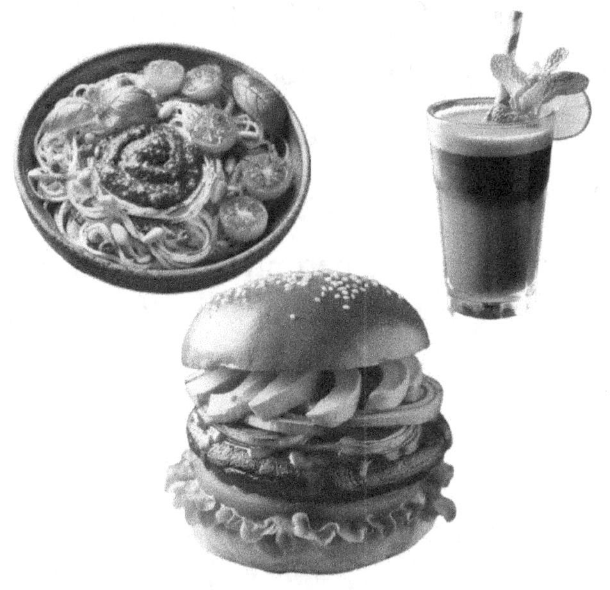

Delicious and Healthy Dishes to Fight Candida and Restore Your Wellness

NOREEN HART

Copyright © 2023 by Noreen Hart

TABLE OF CONTENT

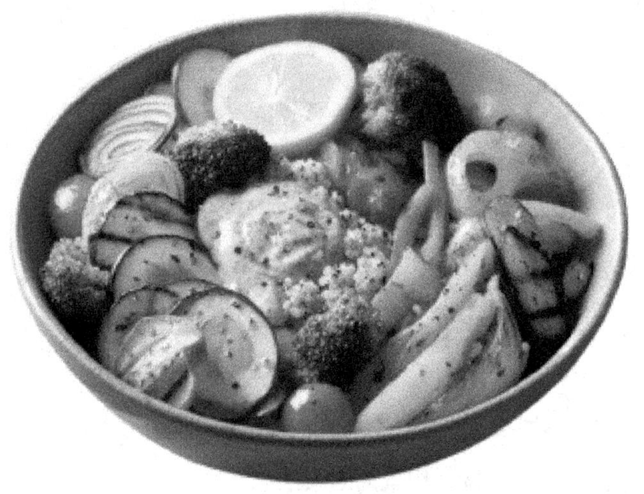

DISCLAIMER

The information provided in this cookbook is intended for general guidance and educational purposes only. It does not substitute professional medical advice, diagnosis, or treatment.

Please consult with a healthcare provider or physician before making any significant changes to your diet, particularly if you have existing medical conditions, allergies, or are taking medication.

The author and publisher are not responsible for any adverse consequences that may arise from implementing the dietary advice, recipes, or information in this book. Always prioritize your health and consult with your healthcare professional on personalized dietary recommendations.

PREFACE

In a world that never seemed to slow down, Emily found herself caught in the endless rush of life. She'd wake up each day feeling tired, her energy reserves sapped, and her spirit weighed down.

Despite her best efforts, she was constantly plagued by nagging sugar cravings, brain fog, and unexplained fatigue.

It was during one of those fatigued afternoons that her life took a pivotal turn. A visit to the hospital for a thorough check-up revealed the culprit behind her relentless exhaustion: Candida overgrowth. Her curiosity piqued, Emily dove into research, eager to understand what was happening within her body.

She soon found herself navigating the maze of Candida-related information. She was drawn to a holistic approach to healing, one that extended beyond conventional medicine.

She embarked on a journey that combined the wisdom of vegan recipes and lifestyle changes, discovering that her dietary choices could play a vital role in her well-being.

As she delved deeper into the subject, Emily uncovered a wealth of vegan recipes that aligned seamlessly with the principles of the Candida Diet.

These recipes, with their enticing flavors and healthful ingredients, quickly became the centerpiece of her daily routine. She experienced a transformation she had never thought possible – her skin cleared, her energy levels soared, and her vitality returned with newfound vigor.

Emily's journey was not without its share of challenges, but her commitment to well-being was unwavering. The secrets to her healing journey were no longer hidden, and she wished for others to discover the transformative potential of a holistic approach to health.

Just like Emily, you too can embark on a life-changing expedition to well-being. This book unveils the secrets that will empower you to transform your health, rekindle your energy, and embrace a life filled with renewed vitality.

Discover the transformative potential of a holistic approach to health, where the wisdom of vegan recipes and lifestyle changes can lead you to a path of balance, wellness, and joy.

Are you ready to step onto the path of wellness and take charge of your Candida journey? Your adventure begins now, and "Candida Diet Cookbook for Vegans" is here to guide you toward a future where Candida is no longer in control, and you are the master of your well-being.

INTRODUCTION

Welcome to "The Candida Diet Cookbook for Vegans." In the journey to better health and wellness, the role of diet is often underestimated.

However, when it comes to candida overgrowth, dietary choices can play a critical role in managing and controlling this common fungal condition.

In this book, we'll explore the Candida Diet, specifically tailored for vegans. Candida overgrowth can lead to a host of uncomfortable symptoms, such as digestive issues, fatigue, and skin problems.

By making informed choices about the foods you consume, you can take control of your health and well-being.

Setting the Stage

Our journey begins with an understanding of candida overgrowth and how it can affect your life. Candida is a type of yeast that naturally resides in your body, primarily in the gut. Under usual circumstances, it shares a harmonious existence with other microorganisms. However, when its balance is disrupted, it can lead to candida overgrowth, which in turn can trigger a range of health issues.

Importance of Diet in Candida Control

Diet plays a pivotal role in managing candida overgrowth. By eliminating foods that nourish candida, such as sugar and refined carbohydrates, and incorporating anti-fungal, vegan-friendly choices, you can help your body regain its balance.

The Candida Diet focuses on creating an environment that hinders candida growth, making it an essential part of your journey to wellness.

What to Expect in This Book

This book is your guide to embracing a vegan lifestyle while effectively managing candida overgrowth. We'll begin by exploring the basics of the Candida Diet, with a detailed breakdown of foods to avoid and those you should include in your diet. I'll also provide you with sample shopping lists to make your transition easier.

As the heart of this book, you'll find a diverse collection of vegan recipes carefully crafted to align with the Candida Diet principles.

Whether you're looking for a satisfying breakfast, a nourishing lunch, a hearty dinner, or a delightful dessert, I've got you covered with mouthwatering recipes that won't compromise your health goals.

Your journey to candida control and a thriving vegan lifestyle starts here. So, let's explore the world of delicious and healthful recipes, armed with the knowledge to make choices that will leave candida in the past and a happier, healthier you in the future.

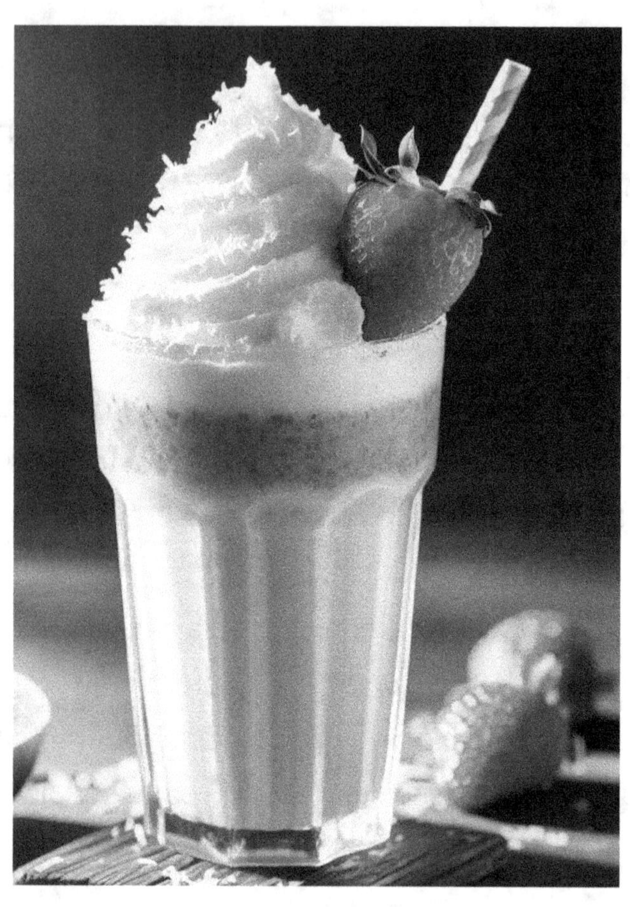

CHAPTER 1

Candida Diet Basics

Understanding the Candida Diet is essential for effectively managing candida overgrowth. In this section, we will explore the key principles of the diet, including the foods you should avoid and those you should include in your daily meals.

Additionally, we will provide you with candida-friendly shopping lists tailored for vegans to help you navigate your grocery trips.

Foods to Avoid

One of the fundamental aspects of the Candida Diet is identifying and avoiding foods that promote candida overgrowth. By eliminating these foods, you create an environment less conducive to candida growth. Here are some primary foods to avoid:

1. Sugar and Sweeteners:

Candida thrives on sugar. Eliminate all forms of refined sugar, honey, maple syrup, and artificial sweeteners from your diet. Opt for stevia or xylitol as healthier sweetener alternatives.

2. Refined Carbohydrates:

Foods like white bread, pasta, and processed cereals quickly break down into sugar, providing an ideal environment for candida. Replace them with whole grains like quinoa, brown rice, and gluten-free oats.

3. Processed Foods:

Processed foods often contain additives, preservatives, and hidden sugars. It's best to steer clear of them and opt for fresh, whole foods.

4. Dairy:

Dairy products can contribute to inflammation and yeast overgrowth. Choose dairy-free alternatives like almond milk, coconut yogurt, and vegan cheese.

5. Alcohol:

Alcohol not only contains sugar but also impairs your immune system's ability to control candida. It's advisable to eliminate alcoholic beverages while on the Candida Diet.

Foods to Include

On the flip side, the Candida Diet encourages the consumption of foods that help prevent candida overgrowth and promote balance in your gut. Here's a selection of foods to add to your daily meals:

1. Non-Starchy Vegetables:

Vegetables like broccoli, kale, spinach, and zucchini are low in sugar and high in essential nutrients. They form the foundation of your diet and support overall health.

2. Plant-Based Proteins:

Legumes, tofu, tempeh, and vegan-friendly protein sources provide the amino acids your body needs without feeding candida.

3. Healthy Fats:

Avocado, olive oil, coconut oil, nuts, and seeds are great sources of healthy fats. These fats are an essential part of your diet and help maintain your energy levels.

4. Herbs and Spices:

Many herbs and spices have anti-fungal properties and can enhance the flavor of your dishes. Garlic, oregano, and cinnamon are known for their candida-fighting potential.

Candida Diet Shopping Lists for Vegans

Transitioning to the Candida Diet as a vegan may seem challenging, but with the right ingredients in your pantry, you'll find it more manageable and enjoyable. Here are sample shopping lists to help you stock up on the essentials:

Pantry Staples:

Non-starchy Vegetables (fresh and frozen): Broccoli, kale, spinach, zucchini, cauliflower, bell peppers, and more.

Plant-Based Proteins: Lentils, chickpeas, black beans, tofu, tempeh, and quinoa.

Healthy Fats: Avocado, extra virgin olive oil, coconut oil, nuts (almonds, walnuts, etc.), and seeds (chia, flax, hemp).

Herbs and Spices: Garlic, oregano, cinnamon, turmeric, basil, thyme, and rosemary.

Vegan Dairy Alternatives: Almond milk, coconut yogurt, and vegan cheese.

Gluten-Free Whole Grains: Brown rice, quinoa, gluten-free oats, and millet.

Sweeteners: Stevia, xylitol, and monk fruit sweetener.

Refrigerator and Freezer:

Fresh Non-Starchy Vegetables: Keep a variety of fresh vegetables such as leafy greens, carrots, and cucumbers in the refrigerator.

Plant-Based Protein: Tofu, tempeh, and other vegan protein sources.

Herbs and Spices: Fresh herbs like basil and thyme, as well as minced garlic and ginger for cooking.

Vegan Dairy Alternatives: Almond milk, coconut yogurt, and any other preferred plant-based dairy.

Fresh Produce:

Avocado
Fresh berries (if desired)
Lemons and limes for zesting and flavoring
Any other fresh produce you enjoy and that aligns with the Candida Diet principles.

Baking Essentials (if desired):

Gluten-free flour like almond flour, coconut flour, or cassava flour.

Baking powder.

Plant-based sweeteners like stevia, xylitol, and monk fruit.

These shopping lists can serve as your starting point for creating Candida-friendly, vegan meals. While shopping, remember to check labels for hidden sugars and processed additives in packaged foods. With these ingredients on hand, you'll be ready to prepare a variety of delicious and healthful meals in line with the Candida Diet.

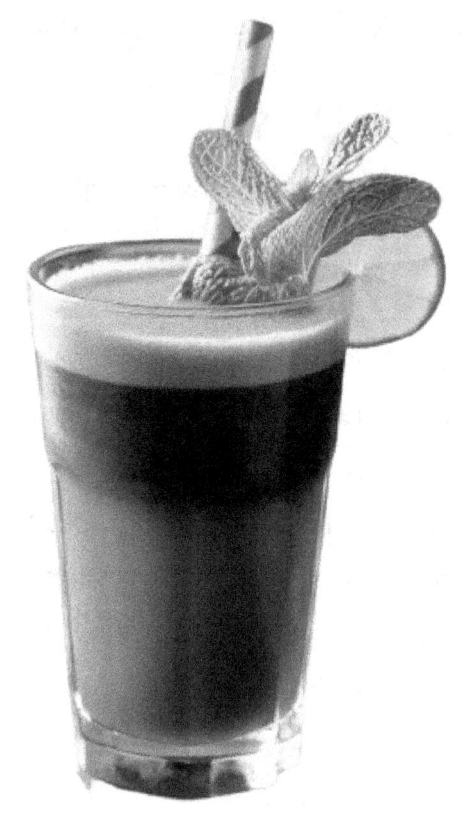

CHAPTER 2

Vegan Breakfast Recipes

1. Vegan Scrambled Tofu

Preparation Time: 15 minutes

Serves: 2

Ingredients:

- 1 block of extra-firm tofu (14 oz)
- 2 tablespoons olive oil
- 1/2 small onion, diced
- 1/2 red bell pepper, diced
- 1/2 green bell pepper, diced
- 1/2 teaspoon turmeric
- 1/2 teaspoon cumin
- Salt and black pepper to taste
- Chives or fresh parsley for garnish (Not compulsory)

Nutritional Information: Calories: 250 per serving, Protein: 16g, Carbohydrates: 8g, Fat: 18g, Fiber: 2g.

Instructions:

1. Begin by gently pressing the tofu to eliminate any excess water. Place the tofu block between paper towels or clean kitchen towels, and gently press with a heavy object for about 10 minutes.

2. Place a big skillet on medium heat, pour in the olive oil, and add the diced onions. Sauté them until they achieve a translucent appearance.

3. Add the diced red and green bell peppers to the skillet and sauté for an additional 3-4 minutes, or until they start to soften.

4. While the vegetables are cooking, crumble the pressed tofu into the skillet. Use a fork or your hands to achieve a scrambled egg-like texture.

5. Sprinkle turmeric and cumin over the crumbled tofu for color and flavor. Add salt and black pepper to your liking for seasoning.

6. Continue cooking, stirring frequently, for about 5-7 minutes, or until the tofu is heated through and has a slightly crispy texture.

7. Taste and adjust seasonings if needed.

8. For extra flavor, consider garnishing with fresh parsley or chives, if desired.

Serving Suggestions:

- Serve the vegan scrambled tofu hot, alongside whole-grain toast, a side of sliced avocado, and a sprinkle of nutritional yeast for a delicious and satisfying breakfast.

2. Savory Oatmeal with Coconut Milk and Vegetables

- **Preparation Time:** 20 minutes
- **Serves:** 2

Ingredients:

- 1 cup rolled oats
- 1 1/2 cups light coconut milk
- 1/2 cup water
- 1/2 teaspoon turmeric
- 1/2 teaspoon cumin
- 1/2 teaspoon paprika

- Salt and black pepper to taste
- 1/2 cup diced mixed vegetables (bell peppers, zucchini, carrots)
- 2 tablespoons chopped fresh cilantro
- 1 tablespoon olive oil

Nutritional Information: Calories: 350 per serving, Protein: 8g, Carbohydrates: 50g, Fat: 13g, Fiber: 6g

Instructions:

1. In a saucepan, combine the rolled oats, light coconut milk, and water. On medium heat, bring the mixture to a boil while stirring occasionally.
2. Once it reaches a boil, reduce the heat to a simmer and add the turmeric, cumin, paprika, salt, and black pepper. Stir well and let it cook for about 5-7 minutes, or until the oats are creamy and tender.
3. While the oats are cooking, heat olive oil in a separate skillet over medium heat. Add the diced mixed vegetables and sauté until they

become tender and slightly caramelized, about 5 minutes.

4. Once the oats are ready, serve them in bowls and top with the sautéed mixed vegetables.

5. Garnish with chopped fresh cilantro.

Serving Suggestions:

- This dish is versatile and pairs well with additional toppings like avocado slices or a sprinkle of nutritional yeast for added flavor and nutrition.

3. Chickpea Flour Pancakes with Coconut Yogurt

- **Preparation Time:** 20 minutes
- **Serves:** 2

Ingredients:

- 1 cup chickpea flour
- 1/2 teaspoon baking powder
- 1/2 teaspoon turmeric
- 1/2 teaspoon cumin

- 1/2 teaspoon paprika
- Salt and black pepper to taste
- 3/4 cup water
- 2 tablespoons chopped fresh cilantro
- 1/2 cup unsweetened coconut yogurt
- Olive oil for cooking

Nutritional Information: Calories: 260 per serving, Protein: 9g, Carbohydrates: 32g, Fat: 11g, Fiber: 7g

Instructions:

1. In a mixing bowl, combine the chickpea flour, baking powder, turmeric, cumin, paprika, salt, and black pepper.
2. Add water gradually and continue to whisk until a smooth batter forms. Stir in chopped fresh cilantro.
3. Heat a non-stick skillet at medium heat, and gently lubricate it with olive oil.
4. Pour a ladle of the chickpea flour batter into the skillet and spread it into a round pancake. Cook for 2-3 minutes on each side until golden

brown and set. Repeat with the remaining batter.

5. Serve the chickpea flour pancakes topped with coconut yogurt.

Serving Suggestions:

- You can also add fresh berries, a drizzle of honey, or a sprinkle of ground flaxseed for extra flavor and nutrition.

4. Happy Gut Bowl

- **Preparation Time:** 15 minutes
- **Serves:** 2

Ingredients:

- 1 cup cooked quinoa
- 1 cup of mixed greens (kale, spinach, arugula, etc.)
- 1/2 cup sauerkraut or fermented vegetables
- 1/2 avocado, sliced
- 1/2 cucumber, diced
- 2 tablespoons pumpkin seeds

- 2 tablespoons tahini dressing (tahini, lemon juice, water, salt)
- A sprinkle of ground flaxseed (optional)

Nutritional Information: Calories: 280 per serving, Protein: 8g, Carbohydrates: 25g, Fat: 18g, Fiber: 7g

Instructions:

1. Start by dividing the cooked quinoa between two serving bowls.
2. Add the mixed greens on top of the quinoa in each bowl.
3. Arrange sauerkraut or fermented vegetables, sliced avocado, and diced cucumber on the greens.
4. Sprinkle pumpkin seeds over the bowls.
5. In a small bowl, mix tahini dressing using tahini, lemon juice, water, and a pinch of salt. Drizzle the dressing over the bowls.
6. Optionally, sprinkle a bit of ground flaxseed for added fiber and omega-3s.

Serving Suggestions:

- Feel free to customize it with your favorite toppings, such as nuts or fresh herbs, to suit your taste.

5. Vegan Omelet with Spinach and Mushrooms

- **Preparation Time:** 20 minutes
- **Serves:** 2

Ingredients:

- 1 cup chickpea flour
- 1/2 teaspoon baking powder
- 1/2 teaspoon turmeric
- 1/2 teaspoon cumin
- Salt and black pepper to taste
- 3/4 cup water
- 1 cup fresh spinach leaves, chopped
- 1 cup sliced mushrooms
- 1/2 small red onion, diced
- Olive oil for cooking

Nutritional Information: Calories: 220 per serving, Protein: 9g, Carbohydrates: 25g, Fat: 10g, Fiber: 5g

Instructions:

1. In a mixing bowl, combine the chickpea flour, baking powder, turmeric, cumin, salt, and black pepper.
2. Add water gradually and continue to whisk until a smooth batter forms.
3. Heat a non-stick skillet at medium heat, and gently lubricate it with olive oil.
4. Pour a portion of the chickpea flour batter into the skillet, swirling it to form a thin omelet.
5. Cook for 2-3 minutes until the omelet is set and the edges start to lift.
6. Sprinkle chopped spinach, sliced mushrooms, and diced red onion on one half of the omelet.
7. Carefully fold the other half of the omelet over the filling to create a half-moon shape.

8. Cook for an additional 2-3 minutes, then carefully flip the omelet and cook for another 2-3 minutes on the other side until both sides are golden brown.

Serving Suggestions:

- This dish pairs well with a side of fresh fruit or a small salad for a balanced morning meal.

6. Coconut Chia Pudding

- **Preparation Time:** 5 minutes (plus 4 hours chilling time)
- **Serves:** 2

Ingredients:

- 1/4 cup chia seeds
- 1 cup unsweetened coconut milk
- 1/2 teaspoon vanilla extract
- 1 tablespoon stevia (or sweetener of choice)

- 1/2 cup mixed fresh berries (blueberries, raspberries, strawberries)
- Shredded coconut for garnish (optional)

Nutritional Information: Calories: 170 per serving, Protein: 4g, Carbohydrates: 16g, Fat: 10g, Fiber: 8g

Instructions:

1. In a mixing bowl, combine chia seeds, unsweetened coconut milk, vanilla extract, and stevia (or your choice of sweetener). Mix well.
2. Cover the bowl and place it in the refrigerator for a minimum of 4 hours or overnight, letting the chia seeds soak up the liquid and develop a pudding-like texture.
3. Once the chia pudding is firm, give it a thorough stir.
4. Divide the pudding into two serving cups or bowls.
5. Top with mixed fresh berries and garnish with shredded coconut if desired.

Serving Suggestions:

- It's a versatile dish, so feel free to customize it with your favorite toppings, such as sliced almonds, a drizzle of honey, or a sprinkle of cinnamon, to suit your taste.

7. Avocado Baked Eggs with Vegetable Hash

- **Preparation Time:** 30 minutes
- **Serves:** 2

Ingredients:

- 1 large avocado
- 2 eggs
- 1/2 cup diced mixed vegetables (bell peppers, zucchini, onions)
- 1/2 teaspoon paprika
- Salt and black pepper to taste
- Fresh parsley for garnish (optional)

Nutritional Information: Calories: 250 per serving, Protein: 11g, Carbohydrates: 12g, Fat: 19g, Fiber: 8g

Instructions:

1. Preheat your oven to 375°F (190°C).
2. Cut the avocados in half and extract the pits.
3. Scoop out some flesh from the center to create a larger cavity for the eggs.
4. Position the avocado halves in a baking dish to stabilize them.
5. In a bowl, combine the diced mixed vegetables, paprika, salt, and black pepper. Mix well.
6. Fill each avocado half with the vegetable mixture, creating a small well in the center for the egg.
7. Crack an egg into each avocado half.
8. Bake in the preheated oven for 15-20 minutes or until the egg whites are set, and the yolks are still slightly runny.
9. Bring it out of the oven and add a touch of fresh parsley, if desired.

Serving Suggestions:

- Pair it with a side of whole-grain toast or a small salad for a complete and satisfying morning meal.

CHAPTER 3

Vegan Lunch Recipes

1. Cauliflower Rice and Vegetable Stir-Fry

- **Preparation Time:** 20 minutes
- **Serves:** 2

Ingredients:

- 1 medium cauliflower head
- 2 tablespoons olive oil
- 1/2 small onion, diced
- 1/2 red bell pepper, sliced
- 1/2 green bell pepper, sliced
- 1 small carrot, thinly sliced
- 1 cup broccoli florets
- 1 cup snap peas or snow peas
- 2 cloves garlic, minced
- 2 tablespoons of low-sodium soy sauce (or tamari, if you want it gluten-free)

- 1 teaspoon ginger, grated
- Salt and black pepper to taste
- Green onions or fresh cilantro for garnish (optional)

Nutritional Information: Calories: 180 per serving, Protein: 6g, Carbohydrates: 17g, Fat: 12g, Fiber: 6g

Instructions:

1. Start by preparing the cauliflower rice. Separate the leaves and stem from the cauliflower head and cut it into florets. Put the florets into a food processor and pulse until they look like rice. Set aside.
2. Heat up the olive oil in a large skillet or wok on medium-high heat.
3. Add the diced onion and sauté for a couple of minutes until it becomes translucent.
4. Stir in the sliced red and green bell peppers, carrot, broccoli florets, snap peas, and minced garlic. Cook for 5-7 minutes, or until the vegetables are tender but still crisp.

5. Add the cauliflower rice to the skillet, along with low-sodium soy sauce (or tamari), grated ginger, salt, and black pepper.
6. Stir-fry the mixture for an additional 5-7 minutes, until the cauliflower rice is tender and the flavors are well combined.
7. Taste and adjust the seasonings if needed.
8. Garnish with fresh cilantro or green onions, if desired.

Serving Suggestions:

- It's a versatile dish that can be enjoyed as is or paired with a protein source of your choice, such as tofu, tempeh, or chickpeas, for added satiety.

2. Vegan Quinoa Salad

- **Preparation Time:** 20 minutes
- **Serves:** 2

Ingredients:

- 1 cup quinoa, cooked and cooled

- 1 cup of mixed vegetables (bell peppers, cherry tomatoes, cucumbers)
- 1/2 cup cooked chickpeas
- 1/4 cup red onion, finely chopped
- 1/4 cup fresh parsley, chopped
- 1/4 cup fresh mint, chopped
- 2 tablespoons olive oil
- Juice of 1 lemon
- Salt and black pepper to taste
- A pinch of red pepper flakes (optional)

Nutritional Information: Calories: 320 per serving, Protein: 10g, Carbohydrates: 50g, Fat: 10g, Fiber: 8g

Instructions:

1. In a large bowl, combine the cooked and cooled quinoa with the mixed vegetables, cooked chickpeas, finely chopped red onion, fresh parsley, and fresh mint.
2. In a separate small bowl, whisk together the olive oil, lemon juice, salt, black pepper, and a pinch of red pepper flakes, if desired.

3. Pour the dressing over the quinoa salad and toss everything to combine.

4. Taste and adjust the seasonings if needed.

5. Allow the salad to sit for a few minutes to let the flavors meld.

Serving Suggestions:

- It's a versatile dish that can be served on its own or alongside a leafy green salad for extra freshness and nutrition.

3. Vegan Zucchini Noodles with Pesto

- **Preparation Time:** 15 minutes
- **Serves:** 2

Ingredients:

- 2 medium zucchinis
- 1 cup fresh basil leaves
- 1/4 cup pine nuts
- 2 cloves garlic
- 1/4 cup nutritional yeast (or vegan Parmesan)

- 1/4 cup extra-virgin olive oil
- Juice of 1 lemon
- Salt and black pepper to taste
- Cherry tomatoes for garnish (optional)

Nutritional Information: Calories: 280 per serving, Protein: 8g, Carbohydrates: 10g, Fat: 24g, Fiber: 4g

Instructions:

1. Using a spiralizer or a julienne peeler, create zucchini noodles from the two medium zucchinis. Transfer the zoodles to a spacious bowl and leave them aside.
2. In a food processor, combine fresh basil leaves, pine nuts, garlic, nutritional yeast (or vegan Parmesan), extra-virgin olive oil, lemon juice, salt, and black pepper.
3. Process the ingredients until you have a creamy pesto sauce.
4. Pour the pesto sauce over the zucchini noodles and toss to coat them thoroughly.
5. Allow the zucchini noodles to marinate in the pesto for a few minutes.

6. Garnish with cherry tomatoes, if desired.

Serving Suggestions:

- You can serve it as is or add extra protein by topping it with roasted chickpeas or tofu for a well-rounded meal.

4. Vegan Sweet Potato and Black Bean Salad

- **Preparation Time:** 30 minutes
- **Serves:** 2

Ingredients:

- 2 medium sweet potatoes, peeled and diced
- 1 can (15 oz) of drained and rinsed black beans
- 1 cup corn kernels (fresh or frozen)
- 1/2 red onion, finely chopped
- 1/4 cup fresh cilantro, chopped
- 1/4 cup lime juice
- 2 tablespoons olive oil
- 1 teaspoon ground cumin

- Salt and black pepper to taste
- Avocado slices for garnish (optional)

Nutritional Information: Calories: 330 per serving, Protein: 9g, Carbohydrates: 58g, Fat: 9g, Fiber: 13g

Instructions:

1. Preheat your oven to 400°F (200°C).
2. In a large mixing bowl, toss the diced sweet potatoes with a drizzle of olive oil, salt, and black pepper.
3. Spread the sweet potato cubes on a baking sheet and roast for about 20-25 minutes, or until they are tender and slightly caramelized.
4. While the sweet potatoes are roasting, in a separate bowl, combine the black beans, corn kernels, finely chopped red onion, and fresh cilantro.
5. In a small bowl, whisk together the lime juice, olive oil, ground cumin, salt, and black pepper to create the dressing.
6. Once the sweet potatoes are ready, add them to the bowl with the bean and corn mixture.

7. Add the dressing to the salad and toss everything to combine evenly.

8. Garnish with avocado slices, if desired.

Serving Suggestions:

- It's a well-balanced dish on its own, but you can also pair it with a side of whole-grain bread or brown rice for added complexity.

5. Vegan Portobello Mushroom Burger

- **Preparation Time:** 30 minutes
- **Serves:** 2

Ingredients:

- 2 large Portobello mushrooms, stems removed
- 1/4 cup balsamic vinegar
- 2 tablespoons olive oil
- 2 cloves garlic, minced
- Salt and black pepper to taste
- 2 whole-grain burger buns
- 2 tablespoons vegan mayonnaise

- 4 lettuce leaves
- 2 tomato slices
- 4 red onion rings
- Dijon mustard for garnish (optional)

Nutritional Information: Calories: 250 per serving, Protein: 6g, Carbohydrates: 32g, Fat: 11g, Fiber: 6g

Instructions:

1. In a shallow dish, whisk together balsamic vinegar, olive oil, minced garlic, salt, and black pepper to create a marinade.
2. Place the Portobello mushrooms in the marinade, making sure they are well-coated. Give them time to marinate for around 10-15 minutes.
3. Get the grill or grill pan ready by preheating it to medium-high heat.
4. Grill the marinated Portobello mushrooms for 5-7 minutes on each side, or until they are tender and have grill marks.

5. While the mushrooms are grilling, toast the whole-grain burger buns on the grill for 1-2 minutes until they are lightly toasted.

6. Assemble the burgers by spreading vegan mayonnaise on the bottom half of each bun.

7. Place a grilled Portobello mushroom on each bun.

8. Top the mushrooms with lettuce leaves, tomato slices, and red onion rings.

9. Optionally, add a drizzle of Dijon mustard for extra flavor.

10. Place the top half of the bun on each burger to complete the assembly.

Serving Suggestions:

- Serve it with a side of sweet potato fries or a simple green salad for a delicious meal.

6. Tofu Salad Sandwich on Gluten-Free Bread

- **Preparation Time:** 20 minutes
- **Serves:** 2

Ingredients:

- 8 oz firm tofu, pressed and cubed
- 2 tablespoons vegan mayonnaise
- 1/2 teaspoon Dijon mustard
- 1/4 cup finely chopped celery
- 1/4 cup finely chopped red bell pepper
- 2 tablespoons red onion, finely chopped
- 2 tablespoons fresh parsley, chopped
- Salt and black pepper to taste
- 4 slices of gluten-free bread
- Lettuce leaves and tomato slices for garnish (optional)

Nutritional Information: Calories: 250 per serving, Protein: 12g, Carbohydrates: 15g, Fat: 16g, Fiber: 2g

Instructions:

1. Begin by gently pressing the tofu to eliminate any excess water. Place the tofu between paper towels or clean kitchen towels and gently press with a heavy object for about 10 minutes.

2. Transfer the pressed tofu into a mixing bowl and break it into small pieces.

3. Add vegan mayonnaise, Dijon mustard, chopped celery, chopped red bell pepper, chopped red onion, and fresh parsley to the crumbled tofu.

4. Mix everything together until the ingredients are well combined.

5. Season the tofu salad with salt and black pepper to taste.

6. Toast the slices of gluten-free bread if desired.

7. Divide the tofu salad evenly between two slices of bread.

8. Optionally, add lettuce leaves and tomato slices for extra freshness.

9. Top with the remaining slices of bread to complete the sandwiches.

Serving Suggestions:

- It pairs well with a side of carrot sticks, cucumber slices, or your favorite gluten-free chips.

7. Southwestern Pasta Salad

- **Preparation Time:** 20 minutes
- **Serves:** 2

Ingredients:

- 2 cups cooked and cooled gluten-free pasta (e.g., penne, fusilli)
- 1 cup black beans, drained and rinsed
- 1 cup corn kernels (fresh or frozen, cooked)
- 1/2 cup diced red bell pepper
- 1/4 cup red onion, finely chopped
- 1/4 cup fresh cilantro, chopped
- 2 tablespoons olive oil
- Juice of 1 lime
- 1 teaspoon ground cumin
- 1/2 teaspoon chili powder
- Salt and black pepper to taste
- Avocado slices for garnish (optional)

Nutritional Information: Calories: 320 per serving, Protein: 9g, Carbohydrates: 56g, Fat: 8g, Fiber: 8g

Instructions:

1. In a large mixing bowl, combine the cooked and cooled gluten-free pasta, black beans, corn kernels, diced red bell pepper, finely chopped red onion, and fresh cilantro.
2. In a small bowl, whisk together olive oil, lime juice, ground cumin, chili powder, salt, and black pepper to create the dressing.
3. Pour the dressing over the pasta salad and toss everything to coat it evenly.
4. Taste and adjust the seasonings if needed.
5. Allow the salad to sit for a few minutes to let the flavors meld.
6. Garnish with avocado slices, if desired.

Serving Suggestions:

- It's perfect on its own, but you can also serve it with a side of tortilla chips or a dollop of vegan sour cream for added texture and taste.

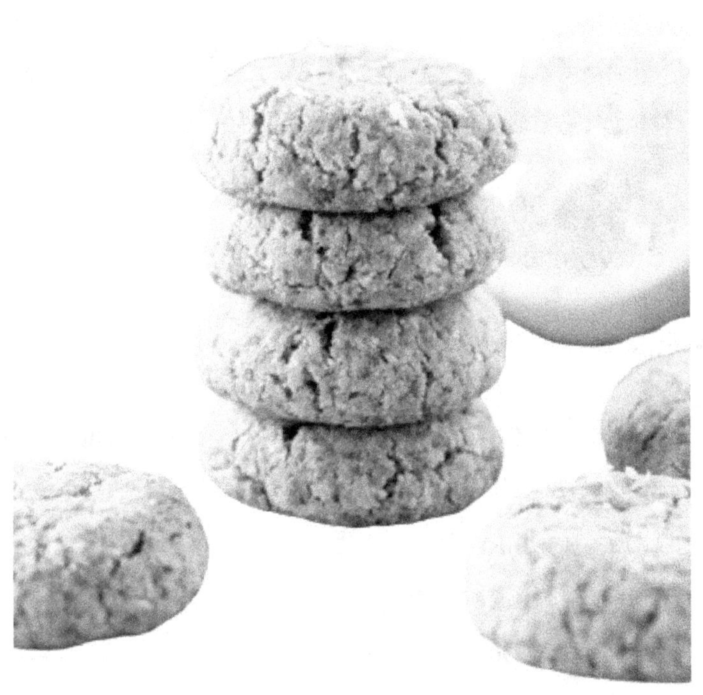

CHAPTER 4

Vegan Dinner Recipes

1. Roasted Vegetable Salad with Tahini Dressing

- **Preparation Time:** 30 minutes
- **Serves:** 2

Ingredients:

- 2 cups of mixed vegetables (e.g., zucchini, bell peppers,, cherry tomatoes)
- 1 cup cauliflower florets
- 1 cup sweet potato, diced
- 2 tablespoons olive oil
- 1 teaspoon ground cumin
- Salt and black pepper to taste
- 1/4 cup tahini
- Juice of 1 lemon
- 2 cloves garlic, minced
- 2 tablespoons fresh parsley, chopped

- Red pepper flakes for garnish (optional)

Nutritional Information: Calories: 320 per serving, Protein: 5g, Carbohydrates: 26g, Fat: 22g, Fiber: 6g

Instructions:

1. Preheat your oven to 400°F (200°C).
2. In a large mixing bowl, toss the mixed vegetables, cauliflower florets, and diced sweet potato with olive oil, ground cumin, salt, and black pepper.
3. Spread the seasoned vegetables on a baking sheet and roast for about 20-25 minutes or until they are tender and slightly caramelized.
4. While the vegetables are roasting, in a small bowl, whisk together tahini, lemon juice, minced garlic, and a pinch of salt to create the dressing.
5. Once the roasted vegetables are ready, transfer them to a serving platter.
6. Drizzle the tahini dressing over the vegetables.
7. Garnish with chopped fresh parsley and a sprinkle of red pepper flakes, if desired.

Serving Suggestions:

- This dish is satisfying on its own, but you can also serve it with a side of quinoa or brown rice for a more substantial meal.

2. Vegan Baked Brussels Sprouts

- **Preparation Time:** 25 minutes
- **Serves:** 2

Ingredients:

- 2 cups Brussels sprouts, trimmed and halved
- 2 tablespoons olive oil
- 2 cloves garlic, minced
- Salt and black pepper to taste
- 1/4 cup nutritional yeast
- 2 tablespoons lemon juice
- 2 tablespoons fresh parsley, chopped
- Lemon zest for garnish (optional)

Nutritional Information: Calories: 150 per serving, Protein: 6g, Carbohydrates: 10g, Fat: 10g, Fiber: 4g

Instructions:

1. Preheat your oven to 400°F (200°C).
2. In a mixing bowl, toss the trimmed and halved Brussels sprouts with olive oil, minced garlic, salt, and black pepper.
3. Lay out the seasoned Brussels sprouts on a baking sheet, ensuring a single layer.
4. Roast in the preheated oven for about 20-25 minutes, or until the sprouts are tender and crispy on the outside, stirring once or twice during cooking.
5. While the Brussels sprouts are roasting, in a small bowl, combine nutritional yeast, lemon juice, and chopped fresh parsley to create the seasoning mixture.
6. Once the Brussels sprouts are ready, transfer them to a serving dish.
7. Sprinkle the nutritional yeast mixture over the roasted Brussels sprouts.
8. Optionally, garnish with lemon zest for an extra zing.

Serving Suggestions:

- They pair well with your favorite grain, such as quinoa or brown rice, and a protein source like tofu or tempeh for a complete meal.

3. Vegan Lentil Stew

- **Preparation Time:** 40 minutes
- **Serves:** 2

Ingredients:

- 1 cup of dried brown or green lentils, rinsed and drained
- 4 cups vegetable broth
- 1 cup diced carrots
- 1 cup diced celery
- 1 cup diced onion
- 2 cloves garlic, minced
- 1 teaspoon ground cumin
- 1/2 teaspoon paprika
- 1/2 teaspoon dried thyme
- Salt and black pepper to taste

- 1 bay leaf
- 1 cup diced tomatoes (canned or fresh)
- 2 cups fresh spinach
- Fresh parsley for garnish (optional)

Nutritional Information: Calories: 350 per serving, Protein: 20g, Carbohydrates: 60g, Fat: 2g, Fiber: 18g

Instructions:

1. In a large pot, combine the rinsed lentils, vegetable broth, diced carrots, diced celery, diced onion, minced garlic, ground cumin, paprika, dried thyme, salt, black pepper, and the bay leaf.
2. Bring the mixture to a boil, then reduce the heat to a simmer and cover the pot. Cook for about 20-25 minutes or until the lentils and vegetables are tender.
3. Stir in the diced tomatoes and fresh spinach.
4. Continue to cook for an additional 5-7 minutes until the spinach wilts, and the stew thickens.
5. Taste and adjust the seasonings if needed.
6. Remove the bay leaf.

Serving Suggestions:

- Serve it with a side of crusty bread or a simple salad for a complete and satisfying meal.

4. Vegan Cilantro Lime Rice with Black Beans

- **Preparation Time:** 30 minutes
- **Serves:** 2

Ingredients:

- 1 cup long-grain white rice (or brown rice for a healthier option)
- 2 cups water
- 1 cup canned black beans, drained and rinsed
- 2 tablespoons fresh cilantro, chopped
- Juice of 1 lime
- Salt and black pepper to taste
- Lime wedges for garnish (optional)

Nutritional Information: Calories: 250 per serving, Protein: 7g, Carbohydrates: 52g, Fat: 1g, Fiber: 6g

Instructions:

1. In a saucepan, combine the rice and water. Bring to a boil, then reduce the heat to low, cover, and simmer for about 15-20 minutes, or until the rice is cooked and the water is absorbed.
2. Fluff the cooked rice with a fork and let it cool slightly.
3. In a mixing bowl, combine the cooked rice, drained black beans, chopped fresh cilantro, and the juice of one lime.
4. Mix everything together until the ingredients are well combined.
5. Add salt and black pepper to your liking for seasoning.

Serving Suggestions:

- It's great as a standalone dish or can be paired with roasted vegetables or a side of guacamole for added flavor and nutrition.

5. Vegan Baked Eggplant Parmesan

- **Preparation Time:** 45 minutes
- **Serves:** 2

Ingredients:

- 1 large eggplant, sliced into 1/2-inch rounds
- 1 cup vegan breadcrumbs
- 1/2 cup vegan Parmesan cheese
- 1 tablespoon dried basil
- 1 tablespoon dried oregano
- Salt and black pepper to taste
- 2 cups marinara sauce
- 1 cup vegan mozzarella cheese, shredded
- Fresh basil leaves for garnish (optional)

Nutritional Information: Calories: 320 per serving, Protein: 12g, Carbohydrates: 45g, Fat: 12g, Fiber: 12g

Instructions:

1. Preheat your oven to 400°F (200°C).

2. In a shallow dish, combine the vegan breadcrumbs, vegan Parmesan cheese, dried basil, dried oregano, salt, and black pepper.

3. Submerge each eggplant slice into the breadcrumb mixture, ensuring that both sides are coated.

4. Place the coated eggplant slices on a baking sheet lined with parchment paper.

5. Bake in the preheated oven for about 20-25 minutes, or until the eggplant slices are tender and golden brown.

6. Add a layer of marinara sauce to a different baking dish.

7. Place half of the baked eggplant slices over the sauce.

8. Sprinkle half of the vegan mozzarella cheese over the eggplant slices.

9. Repeat with the remaining eggplant slices, marinara sauce, and vegan mozzarella cheese.

10. Continue baking for another 15-20 minutes, or until the cheese has melted and is bubbling.

11. Optionally, garnish with fresh basil leaves.

Serving Suggestions:

- It's perfect when served with a side of spaghetti or a fresh green salad for a well-rounded meal.

6. Vegan Spaghetti Squash Primavera

- **Preparation Time:** 45 minutes
- **Serves:** 2

Ingredients:

- 1 medium spaghetti squash
- 2 tablespoons olive oil
- 1/2 red bell pepper, sliced
- 1/2 yellow bell pepper, sliced
- 1/2 zucchini, sliced
- 1/2 yellow squash, sliced
- 1 cup cherry tomatoes, halved
- 2 cloves garlic, minced
- 1 teaspoon dried Italian herbs (e.g., basil, oregano, thyme)
- Salt and black pepper to taste

- Fresh basil leaves for garnish (optional)

Nutritional Information: Calories: 220 per serving, Protein: 4g, Carbohydrates: 28g, Fat: 12g, Fiber: 7g

Instructions:

1. Preheat your oven to 375°F (190°C).
2. Cut the spaghetti squash in half lengthwise and scoop out the seeds and stringy parts.
3. Lay the squash halves on a baking sheet, cut side down.
4. Bake in the preheated oven for about 30-35 minutes, or until the squash flesh is tender and easily shreds into spaghetti-like strands with a fork.
5. While the spaghetti squash is baking, in a large skillet, heat the olive oil over medium heat.
6. Add the sliced red and yellow bell peppers, zucchini, yellow squash, and cherry tomatoes to the skillet. Stir-fry for 5-7 minutes until the vegetables reach a tender state.

7. Stir in the minced garlic, dried Italian herbs, salt, and black pepper. Cook for an additional 2 minutes.

8. Once the spaghetti squash is ready, use a fork to shred the flesh into strands.

9. Add the spaghetti squash strands to the skillet with the sautéed vegetables.

10. Toss everything together to combine.

11. Optionally, garnish with fresh basil leaves.

Serving Suggestions:

- It's perfect on its own, or you can serve it with a side of garlic bread for a complete and satisfying meal.

7. Vegan Cauliflower Alfredo

- **Preparation Time:** 35 minutes
- **Serves:** 2

Ingredients:

- 1 small cauliflower head, cut into florets
- 2 cups vegetable broth

- 1/2 cup unsweetened almond milk
- 2 cloves garlic, minced
- 2 tablespoons nutritional yeast
- 2 tablespoons lemon juice
- Salt and black pepper to taste
- 8 oz whole-grain or gluten-free fettuccine pasta
- Fresh parsley for garnish (optional)

Nutritional Information: Calories: 350 per serving, Protein: 12g, Carbohydrates: 60g, Fat: 5g, Fiber: 9g

Instructions:

1. In a large pot, combine the cauliflower florets and vegetable broth. Bring to a boil, then reduce the heat to simmer and cook for about 10-15 minutes, or until the cauliflower is tender.
2. Using a slotted spoon, remove the cauliflower from the pot and transfer it to a blender or food processor. Reserve the vegetable broth.
3. To the blender or food processor, add the unsweetened almond milk, minced garlic, nutritional yeast, lemon juice, salt, and black pepper.

4. Blend until you achieve a smooth and creamy sauce. If the sauce is too thick, you can add a little of the reserved vegetable broth to achieve your desired consistency.
5. Meanwhile, follow the package instructions to cook the fettuccine pasta. Drain and set aside.
6. In a large mixing bowl, combine the cooked fettuccine pasta with the cauliflower Alfredo sauce. Toss to coat the pasta thoroughly.
7. Optionally, garnish with fresh parsley.

Serving Suggestions:

- It's a delightful dish on its own, but you can also serve it with a side of steamed vegetables or a garden salad for extra freshness and nutrition.

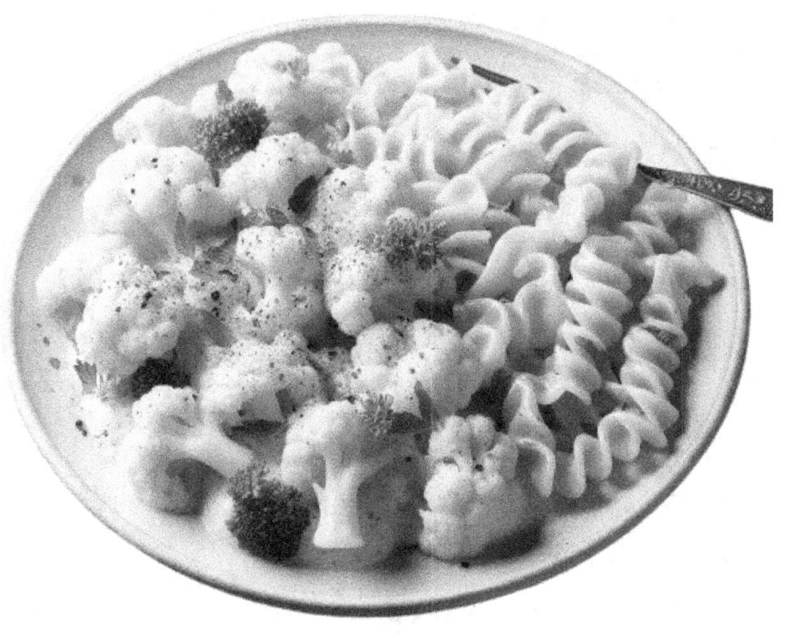

CHAPTER 5

Desserts and Snacks

1. Vegan No-Bake Almond Butter Energy Bites

- **Preparation Time:** 15 minutes
- **Makes:** 12 energy bites

Ingredients:

- 1 cup rolled oats
- 1/2 cup almond butter
- 1/4 cup maple syrup
- 1/4 cup ground flaxseeds
- 1/4 cup vegan chocolate chips
- 1 teaspoon vanilla extract
- A pinch of salt
- Shredded coconut for coating (optional)

Nutritional Information: Calories: 110 per energy bite, Protein: 3g, Carbohydrates: 12g, Fat: 6g, Fiber: 2g

Instructions:

1. In a mixing bowl, combine rolled oats, almond butter, maple syrup, ground flaxseeds, vegan chocolate chips, vanilla extract, and a pinch of salt.
2. Stir your mixture until all the ingredients are thoroughly blended.
3. Place the bowl in the refrigerator for about 15-20 minutes to firm up the mixture, making it easier to handle.
4. Take the mixture out of the refrigerator once the mixture is firm.
5. Using your hands, scoop out small portions of the mixture and roll them into bite-sized balls.
6. If desired, you can roll the energy bites in shredded coconut for added texture and flavor.
7. Place the energy bites on a parchment paper-lined tray or plate.
8. Refrigerate the energy bites for an additional 15 minutes to set.

Serving Suggestions:

- They are perfect for on-the-go snacking or as a quick, sweet treat.

2. Vegan Berry Chia Pudding

- **Preparation Time:** 10 minutes (plus chilling time)
- **Serves:** 2

Ingredients:

- 1/4 cup chia seeds
- 1 cup of unsweetened almond milk (or any of your preferred plant-based milk)
- 1 tablespoon maple syrup (adjust to taste)
- 1/2 teaspoon vanilla extract
- 1 cup of mixed berries (e.g., blueberries, strawberries, raspberries)
- Fresh mint leaves for garnish (optional)

Nutritional Information: Calories: 180 per serving, Protein: 4g, Carbohydrates: 24g, Fat: 8g, Fiber: 10g

Instructions:

1. In a mixing bowl, combine the chia seeds, unsweetened almond milk, maple syrup, and vanilla extract.
2. Stir well to ensure the chia seeds are evenly distributed in the mixture.
3. Let the mixture sit for about 10 minutes, stirring it a few times during this period to prevent clumping.
4. Cover the bowl and refrigerate the chia pudding for at least 2 hours or until it reaches your desired consistency. You can also leave it overnight for a thicker pudding.
5. Before serving, give the chia pudding a good stir to loosen it up and break any clumps.
6. Divide the chia pudding into serving glasses or bowls.
7. Top the chia pudding with mixed berries and fresh mint leaves for a burst of flavor and color.

Serving Suggestions:

- It's a perfect option for a light and fruity treat.

3. Vegan Coconut Yogurt with Berries

- **Preparation Time:** 5 minutes
- **Serves:** 2

Ingredients:

- 1 cup unsweetened coconut yogurt
- 1 cup of mixed berries (e.g., blueberries, strawberries, raspberries)
- 2 tablespoons shredded coconut
- 1 tablespoon maple syrup (adjust to taste)
- Fresh mint leaves for garnish (optional)

Nutritional Information: Calories: 150 per serving, Protein: 4g, Carbohydrates: 20g, Fat: 6g, Fiber: 4g

Instructions:

1. In a mixing bowl, combine unsweetened coconut yogurt and maple syrup.
2. Stir well to sweeten the coconut yogurt to your liking.
3. Divide the sweetened coconut yogurt into serving glasses or bowls.

4. Top each serving with a generous portion of mixed berries.

5. Sprinkle shredded coconut over the berries for added texture and flavor.

6. If desired, you can add a refreshing touch by garnishing it with fresh mint leaves.

Serving Suggestions:

- It's a delightful combination of creamy yogurt and fresh, juicy berries, perfect for a light and refreshing treat.

4. Vegan Zucchini Chips

- **Preparation Time:** 30 minutes
- **Serves:** 2

Ingredients:

- 2 medium zucchinis, thinly sliced
- 2 tablespoons olive oil
- 1/4 cup almond meal (or any flour of your choice)
- 2 tablespoons nutritional yeast

- 1/2 teaspoon garlic powder
- 1/2 teaspoon paprika
- Salt and black pepper to taste
- Cooking spray or parchment paper for baking

Nutritional Information: Calories: 150 per serving, Protein: 5g, Carbohydrates: 7g, Fat: 11g, Fiber: 3g

Instructions:

1. Preheat your oven to 425°F (220°C). Place a wire rack on a baking sheet and lightly coat it with cooking spray or line the baking sheet with parchment paper.

2. In a shallow dish, combine almond meal, nutritional yeast, garlic powder, paprika, salt, and black pepper.

3. Dip each zucchini slice in olive oil, ensuring it's coated evenly, then dredge it in the almond meal mixture, pressing the mixture onto the zucchini to adhere.

4. Place the coated zucchini slices on the prepared wire rack or parchment paper-lined baking sheet.

5. Bake in the preheated oven for about 15-20 minutes, or until the zucchini chips are golden brown and crispy, flipping them halfway through the cooking time.

6. Remove the zucchini chips from the oven and let them cool for a few minutes before serving.

Serving Suggestions:

- They are a delightful alternative to traditional potato chips and pair well with your favorite dipping sauce or vegan ranch dressing.

5. Lemon Coconut Cookies

- **Preparation Time:** 25 minutes
- **Baking Time:** 12-15 minutes
- **Serves:** 2

Ingredients:

- 1 cup almond flour
- 1/2 cup unsweetened shredded coconut
- 2 tablespoons coconut oil, melted
- 2 tablespoons maple syrup

- 1 tablespoon lemon zest
- 2 tablespoons lemon juice
- 1/2 teaspoon vanilla extract
- A pinch of salt

Nutritional Information: Calories: 180 per serving, Protein: 3g, Carbohydrates: 9g, Fat: 15g, Fiber: 3g

Instructions:

1. Preheat your oven to 350°F (175°C). Use parchment paper to line a baking sheet.
2. In a mixing bowl, combine almond flour, unsweetened shredded coconut, melted coconut oil, maple syrup, lemon zest, lemon juice, vanilla extract, and a pinch of salt.
3. Mix the ingredients until a sticky cookie dough forms.
4. Use your hands to shape the dough into small cookie-sized rounds and place them on the prepared baking sheet.
5. Use a fork to gently flatten each cookie and create a crisscross pattern on top.

6. Bake in the preheated oven for 12-15 minutes or until the cookies are lightly golden around the edges.

7. Take the cookies out of the oven and allow them to cool on the baking sheet for a few minutes. As they cool down, they will become firmer.

Serving Suggestions:

- These cookies are perfect with a cup of herbal tea or alongside a glass of almond milk.

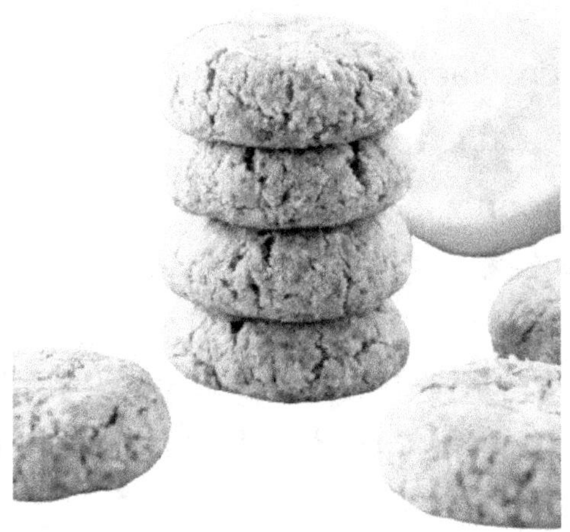

CHAPTER 6

Vegan Smoothies/Drinks

1. Strawberry Coconut Smoothie

- **Preparation Time:** 10 minutes
- **Serves:** 2

Ingredients:

- 1 cup frozen strawberries
- 1/2 cup unsweetened coconut milk
- 1/2 cup plain vegan yogurt
- 1/4 cup unsweetened applesauce
- 1 tablespoon maple syrup (adjust to taste)
- 1/2 teaspoon vanilla extract
- Shredded coconut for garnish (optional)

Nutritional Information: Calories: 150 per serving, Protein: 3g, Carbohydrates: 28g, Fat: 5g, Fiber: 4g

Instructions:

1. In a blender, combine frozen strawberries, unsweetened coconut milk, plain vegan yogurt, unsweetened applesauce, maple syrup, and vanilla extract.

2. Blend until you reach a smooth and creamy texture with all the ingredients. After tasting, you can adjust the sweetness by adding more maple syrup if needed.

3. Pour the strawberry coconut smoothie into glasses.

4. Optionally, garnish with shredded coconut for extra flavor and texture.

Serving Suggestions:

- It's a delightful choice for a quick and nutritious breakfast or a cooling beverage on a warm day.

2. Fresh Basil Iced Tea

- **Preparation Time:** 15 minutes (plus chilling time)
- **Serves:** 2

Ingredients:

- 4 cups water
- 1/4 cup fresh basil leaves
- 2 tablespoons fresh lemon juice
- 1 tablespoon maple syrup (adjust to taste)
- Lemon slices for garnish (optional)

Nutritional Information: Calories: 10 per serving, Carbohydrates: 2g

Instructions:

1. In a saucepan, bring 4 cups of water to a boil.
2. Remove the saucepan from heat and add fresh basil leaves to the hot water.
3. Let the basil steep in the hot water for about 10 minutes to infuse its flavor. You can adjust the

steeping time to achieve your desired basil flavor.

4. Strain the basil-infused water into a pitcher, discarding the basil leaves.
5. Add fresh lemon juice and maple syrup to the pitcher, and stir well.
6. Allow the iced tea to cool to room temperature, then refrigerate for at least 1-2 hours to chill.
7. Serve the Fresh Basil Iced Tea over ice and optionally garnish with lemon slices.

Serving Suggestions:

- It's a perfect choice for a summer day or as a light and flavorful drink to accompany your meals.

3. Beet and Carrot Juice

- **Preparation Time:** 10 minutes
- **Serves:** 2

Ingredients:

- 2 medium beets, peeled and chopped

- 4 large carrots, peeled and chopped
- 1 small apple, cored and chopped
- 1-inch piece of fresh ginger
- 1/2 lemon, peeled
- Fresh mint leaves for garnish (optional)

Nutritional Information: Calories: 80 per serving, Carbohydrates: 20g

Instructions:

1. Wash, peel, and chop the beets, carrots, and apple into smaller pieces, making them easier to juice.

2. In a juicer, process the chopped beets, carrots, apple, fresh ginger, and peeled lemon.

3. Collect the fresh juice in a pitcher or glass.

4. Stir the juice gently to combine all the flavors.

5. Optionally, garnish with fresh mint leaves for extra freshness.

Serving Suggestions:

- It's an excellent choice for a natural energy boost or as a part of your daily intake of vitamins and minerals.

4. Green Detox Smoothie

- **Preparation Time:** 10 minutes
- **Serves:** 2

Ingredients:

- 1 cup fresh spinach leaves
- 1 cup kale leaves, stems removed
- 1/2 cucumber, peeled and chopped
- 1/2 green apple, cored and chopped
- 1/2 lemon, peeled and seeded
- 1 cup of unsweetened almond milk (or any of your preferred plant-based milk)
- 1 tablespoon fresh mint leaves
- 1 teaspoon chia seeds (optional)
- Ice cubes (optional)

Nutritional Information: Calories: 60 per serving, Protein: 2g, Carbohydrates: 12g, Fat: 2g, Fiber: 4g

Instructions:

1. In a blender, combine fresh spinach leaves, kale leaves, peeled cucumber, chopped green apple, peeled lemon, unsweetened almond milk, and fresh mint leaves.
2. If desired, add chia seeds for added fiber and nutrients.
3. Blend until all the ingredients are smooth and the smoothie is a vibrant green color.
4. If you prefer a colder smoothie, you can add a few ice cubes and blend until they're fully incorporated.
5. Pour the Green Detox Smoothie into glasses and serve immediately.

Serving Suggestions:

- It's a fantastic choice for detoxifying and energizing your body while enjoying a burst of natural flavors and vitamins.

5. Cucumber Mint Cooler

- **Preparation Time:** 10 minutes
- **Serves:** 2

Ingredients:

- 1 cucumber, peeled and sliced
- 2 tablespoons fresh mint leaves
- 1 lime, juiced
- 1 tablespoon of maple syrup or honey (adjust to taste)
- 2 cups cold water
- Ice cubes
- Cucumber slices and fresh mint leaves for garnish (optional)

Nutritional Information: Calories: 40 per serving, Carbohydrates: 10g

Instructions:

1. In a blender, combine peeled and sliced cucumber, fresh mint leaves, lime juice, and honey (or maple syrup).

2. Blend the ingredients until you have a smooth and well-mixed mixture.

3. In a pitcher, combine the cucumber-mint mixture with cold water and stir.

4. Fill two glasses with ice cubes.

5. Pour the Cucumber Mint Cooler into the glasses.

6. Optionally, garnish with cucumber slices and fresh mint leaves for an extra refreshing touch.

Serving Suggestions:

- Enjoy the Cucumber Mint Cooler as a cooling and revitalizing drink. It's a great choice to stay hydrated on a hot day or as a healthy alternative to sugary beverages.

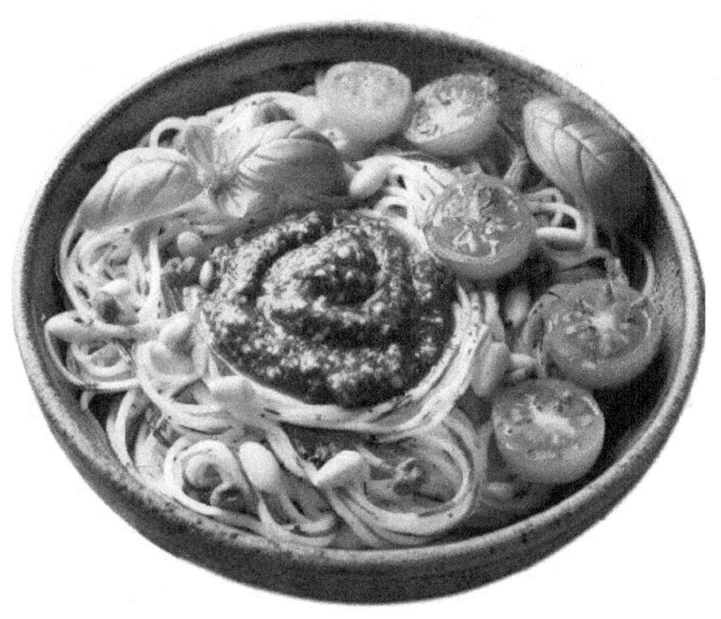

CHAPTER 7

28-Day Meal Plan Sample

Please note that the provided meal plan is a sample and should not be interpreted as a recommendation to consume all the listed recipes in a single day.

The purpose of this meal plan is to offer inspiration and guidance for healthy meal preparation. Feel free to customize this plan further to suit your preferences and dietary requirements.

Day 1:

- Breakfast: Vegan Scrambled Tofu
- Lunch: Cauliflower Rice and Vegetable Stir-Fry
- Dinner: Roasted Vegetable Salad with Tahini Dressing
- Snack: Vegan No-Bake Almond Butter Energy Bites
- Smoothie: Strawberry Coconut Smoothie

Day 2:

- Breakfast: Savory Oatmeal with Coconut Milk and Vegetables
- Lunch: Vegan Quinoa Salad
- Dinner: Vegan Baked Brussels Sprouts
- Snack: Vegan Berry Chia Pudding
- Smoothie: Fresh Basil Iced Tea

Day 3:

- Breakfast: Chickpea Flour Pancakes with Coconut Yogurt
- Lunch: Vegan Zucchini Noodles with Pesto
- Dinner: Vegan Lentil Stew
- Snack: Vegan Coconut Yogurt with Berries
- Smoothie: Beet and Carrot Juice

Day 4:

- Breakfast: Happy Gut Bowl
- Lunch: Vegan Sweet Potato and Black Bean Salad

- Dinner: Vegan Cilantro Lime Rice with Black Beans
- Snack: Vegan Zucchini Chips
- Smoothie: Green Detox Smoothie

Day 5:

- Breakfast: Vegan Omelette with Spinach and Mushrooms
- Lunch: Vegan Portobello Mushroom Burger
- Dinner: Vegan Baked Eggplant Parmesan
- Snack: Lemon Coconut Cookies
- Smoothie: Cucumber Mint Cooler

Day 6:

- Breakfast: Coconut Chia Pudding
- Lunch: Tofu Salad Sandwich on Gluten-Free Bread
- Dinner: Vegan Spaghetti Squash Primavera
- Snack: Vegan No-Bake Almond Butter Energy Bites

Day 7:

- Breakfast: Avocado Baked Eggs with Vegetable Hash
- Lunch: Southwestern Pasta Salad
- Dinner: Vegan Cauliflower Alfredo
- Snack: Vegan Berry Chia Pudding

Day 8:

- Breakfast: Savory Oatmeal with Coconut Milk and Vegetables
- Lunch: Chickpea Flour Pancakes with Coconut Yogurt
- Dinner: Vegan Baked Brussels Sprouts
- Snack: Vegan Coconut Yogurt with Berries
- Smoothie: Strawberry Coconut Smoothie

Day 9:

- Breakfast: Vegan Sweet Potato and Black Bean Salad
- Lunch: Vegan Zucchini Noodles with Pesto
- Dinner: Happy Gut Bowl

- Snack: Vegan Zucchini Chips
- Smoothie: Fresh Basil Iced Tea

Day 10:

- Breakfast: Vegan Omelette with Spinach and Mushrooms
- Lunch: Roasted Vegetable Salad with Tahini Dressing
- Dinner: Vegan Spaghetti Squash Primavera
- Snack: Lemon Coconut Cookies
- Smoothie: Beet and Carrot Juice

Day 11:

- Breakfast: Coconut Chia Pudding
- Lunch: Tofu Salad Sandwich on Gluten-Free Bread
- Dinner: Vegan Lentil Stew
- Snack: Vegan Berry Chia Pudding
- Smoothie: Green Detox Smoothie

Day 12:

- Breakfast: Avocado Baked Eggs with Vegetable Hash
- Lunch: Southwestern Pasta Salad
- Dinner: Vegan Baked Eggplant Parmesan
- Snack: Vegan No-Bake Almond Butter Energy Bites
- Smoothie: Cucumber Mint Cooler

Day 13:

- Breakfast: Savory Oatmeal with Coconut Milk and Vegetables
- Lunch: Vegan Quinoa Salad
- Dinner: Vegan Baked Brussels Sprouts
- Snack: Vegan Coconut Yogurt with Berries
- Smoothie: Strawberry Coconut Smoothie

Day 14:

- Breakfast: Chickpea Flour Pancakes with Coconut Yogurt
- Lunch: Vegan Zucchini Noodles with Pesto

- Dinner: Vegan Cilantro Lime Rice with Black Beans
- Snack: Vegan Zucchini Chips
- Smoothie: Fresh Basil Iced Tea

Day 15:

- Breakfast: Vegan Sweet Potato and Black Bean Salad
- Lunch: Vegan Cauliflower Alfredo
- Dinner: Roasted Vegetable Salad with Tahini Dressing
- Snack: Vegan No-Bake Almond Butter Energy Bites
- Smoothie: Green Detox Smoothie

Day 16:

- Breakfast: Vegan Scrambled Tofu
- Lunch: Vegan Quinoa Salad
- Dinner: Vegan Baked Brussels Sprouts
- Snack: Vegan Berry Chia Pudding
- Smoothie: Cucumber Mint Cooler

Day 17:

- Breakfast: Chickpea Flour Pancakes with Coconut Yogurt
- Lunch: Vegan Zucchini Noodles with Pesto
- Dinner: Vegan Lentil Stew
- Snack: Vegan Coconut Yogurt with Berries
- Smoothie: Beet and Carrot Juice

Day 18:

- Breakfast: Happy Gut Bowl
- Lunch: Vegan Sweet Potato and Black Bean Salad
- Dinner: Vegan Cilantro Lime Rice with Black Beans
- Snack: Vegan Zucchini Chips
- Smoothie: Strawberry Coconut Smoothie

Day 19:

- Breakfast: Vegan Omelette with Spinach and Mushrooms
- Lunch: Vegan Portobello Mushroom Burger

- Dinner: Vegan Baked Eggplant Parmesan
- Snack: Lemon Coconut Cookies
- Smoothie: Fresh Basil Iced Tea

Day 20:

- Breakfast: Coconut Chia Pudding
- Lunch: Tofu Salad Sandwich on Gluten-Free Bread
- Dinner: Vegan Spaghetti Squash Primavera
- Snack: Vegan No-Bake Almond Butter Energy Bites
- Smoothie: Avocado Smoothie

Day 21:

- Breakfast: Avocado Baked Eggs with Vegetable Hash
- Lunch: Southwestern Pasta Salad
- Dinner: Vegan Cauliflower Alfredo
- Snack: Vegan Berry Chia Pudding
- Smoothie: Mango Ginger Smoothie

Day 22:

- Breakfast: Savory Oatmeal with Coconut Milk and Vegetables
- Lunch: Chickpea Flour Pancakes with Coconut Yogurt
- Dinner: Vegan Baked Brussels Sprouts
- Snack: Vegan Coconut Yogurt with Berries
- Smoothie: Green Detox Smoothie

Day 23:

- Breakfast: Vegan Sweet Potato and Black Bean Salad
- Lunch: Vegan Zucchini Noodles with Pesto
- Dinner: Happy Gut Bowl
- Snack: Vegan Zucchini Chips
- Smoothie: Strawberry Coconut Smoothie

Day 24:

- Breakfast: Vegan Omelette with Spinach and Mushrooms

- Lunch: Roasted Vegetable Salad with Tahini Dressing
- Dinner: Vegan Spaghetti Squash Primavera
- Snack: Lemon Coconut Cookies
- Smoothie: Fresh Basil Iced Tea

Day 25:

- Breakfast: Coconut Chia Pudding
- Lunch: Tofu Salad Sandwich on Gluten-Free Bread
- Dinner: Vegan Lentil Stew
- Snack: Vegan Berry Chia Pudding
- Smoothie: Beet and Carrot Juice

Day 26:

- Breakfast: Avocado Baked Eggs with Vegetable Hash
- Lunch: Southwestern Pasta Salad
- Dinner: Vegan Baked Eggplant Parmesan
- Snack: Vegan No-Bake Almond Butter Energy Bites
- Smoothie: Cucumber Mint Cooler

Day 27:

- Breakfast: Savory Oatmeal with Coconut Milk and Vegetables
- Lunch: Vegan Quinoa Salad
- Dinner: Vegan Baked Brussels Sprouts
- Snack: Vegan Coconut Yogurt with Berries
- Smoothie: Strawberry Coconut Smoothie

Day 28:

- Breakfast: Chickpea Flour Pancakes with Coconut Yogurt
- Lunch: Vegan Zucchini Noodles with Pesto
- Dinner: Vegan Cilantro Lime Rice with Black Beans
- Snack: Vegan Zucchini Chips
- Smoothie: Fresh Basil Iced Tea

CHAPTER 8

Conclusion

In the journey to manage Candida overgrowth through a vegan diet, it's important to reflect on the core principles that have guided us in this endeavor. We've explored the Candida Diet Basics, including foods to avoid and those to include, and we've delved into the specifics of Candida Diet shopping for vegans.

As we conclude our exploration, let's recap the key takeaways, discuss the importance of achieving balance and wellness, and leave you with some final thoughts and encouragement.

Recap of Candida Diet Basics

Our journey began by understanding the foundation of the Candida Diet. We've learned to be mindful of the foods to avoid, such as sugary treats, refined carbohydrates, and yeast-containing products.

Instead, we embraced a variety of vegan-friendly foods, including non-starchy vegetables, plant-based proteins, and gluten-free grains. We also recognized the significance of planning our meals meticulously, ensuring that we maintain the Candida Diet's integrity while enjoying a diverse and nutritious diet.

Achieving Balance and Wellness

Balancing the Candida Diet with your overall wellness is paramount. While the diet plays a crucial role in managing Candida overgrowth, it is equally important to consider your general well-being.

Staying physically active and managing stress are integral components of a holistic approach to health. Incorporating relaxation techniques, such as yoga or meditation, into your daily routine can significantly contribute to a balanced and calm state of mind.

Final Thoughts and Encouragement

The journey to balance your health and manage Candida overgrowth through a vegan diet may present its challenges, but it's important to remember that you're not alone in this endeavor.

There's a wealth of resources, support, and delicious recipes at your disposal to guide you through your Candida Diet journey. The commitment to your health is an investment in your well-being that will reward you with vitality and resilience.

It's essential to acknowledge that maintaining a Candida Diet can sometimes be challenging, especially when faced with tempting foods that are off-limits.

In these moments, remember the progress you've made, the positive changes in your health, and the immense potential for a vibrant future.

Above all, approach your journey with self-compassion and patience. Health is a lifelong endeavor, and every small step you take toward maintaining balance contributes to your overall well-being.

In closing, our exploration of the Candida Diet for vegans is a testament to your dedication to achieving optimal health and vitality. It's a journey that empowers you to make mindful choices, savor nourishing meals, and celebrate the synergy of a vegan lifestyle and Candida management.

As you continue on your path to wellness, remember that each day is an opportunity for progress and personal growth. Embrace the delicious recipes, make room for mindfulness, and nourish your body and spirit.

Together, we've unlocked the potential for balanced health and vitality, and the future is filled with opportunities to thrive.

Thank you for embarking on this journey to better health through the Candida Diet for vegans. Your commitment and determination are the keys to your success, and may your path be filled with vibrant well-being, joy, and fulfillment.